DASH Diet Made Easy

25 DASH Diet Recipes for Beginners!

Table of Contents

INTRODUCTION

I want to thank you for choosing this book, *'DASH Diet Made Easy - 25 DASH Diet Recipes for Beginners!'*

Do you want to live a healthier life and avoid problems like high blood pressure, diabetes and a couple of forms of cancer? Then DASH diet is the best option that's available for you.

DASH stands for **D**ietary **A**pproach to **S**top **H**ypertension. This diet is especially designed for preventing and controlling high blood pressure levels. On this diet, the amount of sodium you consume is controlled. Instead of this, you will need to consume foods that are rich in nutrients like vitamins and important minerals like potassium, magnesium and calcium. This isn't just a diet, but it is a lifestyle. By simply following this diet, you will notice that your blood pressure will decrease by two points within the first couple of weeks. Over a period of time, you will notice a reduction in your systolic blood pressure by about eight to fourteen points!

This diet promotes a healthy way of eating and has multiple health benefits apart from lowering your blood pressure. The DASH diet can help in preventing certain diseases like osteoporosis, cancer, heart diseases, stroke and diabetes as well.

In this book, you will find 25 DASH-friendly recipes that you can make use of for reducing and controlling your high blood pressure within a few days. Over a period of few weeks, you will see a significant change in your overall health. These recipes will not only help you in reducing your risk of certain diseases but will also help you in cutting down on your weight and maintain the weight loss as well.

So, all that is left for you to do is get started!

Chapter 1: DASH Diet Breakfast Recipes

1. Cranberry Orange Muffins

Serves: 8

Ingredients:

- ½ cup non-fat Plain Greek yogurt
- 1 egg
- 2 tablespoons canola oil
- 1 tablespoon orange zest, grated
- ½ cup + 6 tablespoons all-purpose flour
- ½ teaspoon baking powder
- 2 tablespoons flaxseed meal
- ½ teaspoon baking soda
- ¼ teaspoon ground cinnamon
- ½ cup sugar
- 2 tablespoons brown sugar
- 1 tablespoon orange juice concentrate
- 1 teaspoon vanilla extract
- ¼ teaspoon salt
- ¾ cup cranberries, fresh or frozen

Method:

1. Grease muffin cups or a muffin tin with a little oil or butter. Place a paper cup liner in each.
2. Add sugar, yogurt, oil, egg, orange juice, vanilla and orange zest into a bowl. Stir.
3. Add flour, flaxseed, baking powder, baking soda, cinnamon and salt into another bowl.
4. Add the dry ingredients into the bowl of wet ingredients.

Beat with an electric mixer on low speed until well combined.

5. Add cranberries and fold gently.
6. Pour the batter into the prepared muffin tins.
7. Place the muffin tin in a preheated oven and bake at 350 F for about 22 minutes or until a toothpick when inserted in the center comes out clean and the top is golden brown.

2. Stuffed French Toast

Serves: 4

Ingredients:

- ¼ cup fat free cream cheese
- 4 slices French bread (1 inch thick)
- 1 small egg, lightly beaten
- 1 egg white
- 6 tablespoons fat free milk
- 1/8 teaspoon apple pie spice
- ¼ + 1 tablespoon cup strawberry or apricot spreadable fruit
- ¼ teaspoon vanilla extract
- Nonstick cooking spray

Method:

1. Add cream cheese and 1-tablespoon strawberry or apricot spreadable fruit into a bowl and mix well.
2. Make pockets in slices of bread using a serrated knife. Make the cut half way along the length.
3. Spoon about a tablespoon of the cream cheese mixture in each bread pocket.
4. Add white, egg, milk, apple pie spice and vanilla into a bowl and whisk well.
5. Place a nonstick griddle over medium heat. Spray the griddle with cooking spray.
6. Dip a bread pocket in the egg mixture and immediately take it out and place on the heated griddle.
7. Cook until golden brown on the bottom side. Flip sides and cook the other side too.
8. Repeat with the remaining bread pockets.

9. Add remaining spreadable strawberry into a saucepan and place over medium heat. When it melts, remove from heat.
10. Spread over the French toast and serve.

Don't forget to like this book and leave a review here: https://www.amazon.com/DASH-Diet-Made-Easy-Beginners-ebook/dp/B071GRN2CV

3. Southwestern Breakfast Bake

Serves: 12

Ingredients:

- 1 ½ cans (15 ounces each) black beans, rinsed, drained
- 3 cans (4 ½ ounces each) diced green chili peppers, drained
- Hot pepper sauce (optional)
- 1 ½ cups sharp cheddar cheese
- 6 ounces Monterey Jack cheese with jalapeño peppers
- 5 eggs, separated
- 3 tablespoons all-purpose flour
- ¾ cup milk
- Sour cream, as required (optional)
- 1 ¼ cups enchilada sauce
- ¾ cup green onions, thinly sliced
- 3 cloves garlic, minced
- ½ teaspoon salt or to taste
- 2 tablespoons fresh cilantro, chopped
- Salsa to serve (optional)

Method:

1. Grease a baking dish with a little oil.
2. Add black beans, enchilada sauce, green onions, green chili peppers, hot pepper sauce and garlic. Mix well. Top with cheese.
3. Beat whites with an electric mixer until soft peaks are formed.
4. Add yolks into another bowl and whisk with a wire whisk. Add flour and salt and whisk again.
5. Add milk and whisk until smooth. Add the whites and

fold gently.

6. Pour this mixture over the cheese layer in the baking dish.
7. Bake in a preheated oven at 325 F for about 45 minutes or until the eggs are set.
8. When done, let it remain in the oven for 15-20 minutes.
9. Garnish with cilantro and serve with salsa.

4. Poblano Tofu Scramble

Serves: 2

Ingredients:

- 8-9 ounces extra firm water packed tofu, drained, pat dried, crumbled
- 1 fresh poblano chili pepper, deseeded, chopped
- 1 clove garlic, minced
- ¼ teaspoon ground cumin
- ¼ teaspoon salt or to taste
- ½ cup plum tomatoes, deseeded, chopped
- 2 teaspoons olive oil
- 1 small onion, chopped
- ½ teaspoon chili powder
- ¼ teaspoon dried oregano, crushed
- 2 teaspoons lime juice
- Fresh cilantro, chopped to serve

Method:

1. Place a nonstick skillet over medium high heat. Add oil. When the oil is heated, add chili pepper, garlic and onion and sauté for a few minutes until the onions are translucent.
2. Add chili powder, salt and cumin and sauté for a few seconds until fragrant.
3. Add tofu and stir.
4. Lower heat and cook until thoroughly heated. Stir occasionally.
5. Add lime juice and tomatoes and stir.
6. Serve immediately garnished with cilantro.

Chapter 2: DASH Diet Appetizer Recipes

5. Southwestern Potato Skin

Serves: 6

Ingredients:

- 3 large baking potatoes, scrubbed
- ½ teaspoon chili powder
- 3 slices turkey bacon, cooked until crispy, chopped
- 1 green onion, thinly sliced
- 1 teaspoon olive oil
- Hot pepper sauce to taste
- 1 small tomato, chopped
- ¼ cup cheddar cheese, shredded

Method:

1. Prick the potatoes all over with a fork.
2. Place in the microwave and cook on high for about 10 minutes or until tender.
3. Place the potatoes on a wire rack to cool. When cool enough to handle, halve the potatoes lengthwise and make potato cases by scooping some of the flesh from the middle. Leave about ¼ inch of the potato flesh on all the sides. Use the scooped potato for some other recipe.
4. Add oil, chili powder and hot sauce into a bowl and mix well. Brush this mixture on the inside of the potato cases.
5. Add bacon, tomato and onions into a bowl and mix well. Stuff this mixture in the potato cases and place on a baking sheet. Sprinkle cheese all over the stuffing.
6. Bake in a preheated oven at 450 F for 8-10 minutes or

until the cheese melts.

7. Serve immediately.

6. Grilled Pineapple

Serves: 4

Ingredients:

For the marinade:

- 1 tablespoon dark honey
- 2 teaspoons lime juice
- 1/8 teaspoon ground cloves
- ½ tablespoon olive oil
- ½ teaspoon ground cinnamon

For the pineapple:

- 1 medium ripe pineapple, peeled, chopped into chunks
- ½ tablespoon lime zest, grated
- ½ tablespoon dark rum, optional
- 4 wooden skewers soaked in water for 30 minutes or use metal skewers

Method:

1. Preheat a grill or a broiler. Grease the grill rack or broiler pan with cooking spray.
2. Place the rack about 6 inches away from the heating source.
3. Add all the ingredients of the marinade in a bowl and whisk well.
4. Brush the pineapple with the marinade. Place on the grill and grill until golden brown.
5. Baste with the marinade a couple of times while it is grilling.

6. Place the grilled pineapple on a serving platter. Brush with rum. Garnish with lime zest and serve hot or warm.

7. Shrimp Ceviche

Serves: 4

Ingredients:

- ¼ pound raw shrimp, cut into ¼ inch pieces
- 1 teaspoon ground cumin
- Juice of a lime
- Zest of a lime, grated
- Juice of a lemon
- Zest of a lemon, grated
- 1 medium red onion, chopped
- 1 tablespoon garlic, minced
- 2 tablespoons Serrano chili pepper, deseeded, chopped
- 2 tablespoons fresh cilantro, chopped
- ½ cup tomato, diced
- 1 tablespoon olive oil
- ½ cup black beans, cooked
- ½ cup cucumber, peeled, diced

Method:

1. Add shrimp into a bowl. Pour lemon juice and lime juice over it. Cover and refrigerate for at least 3-4 hours or until the shrimp turns white and is firm to touch.
2. Add rest of the ingredients into a bowl. Mix well. Add the cold shrimp into it and toss.
3. Serve with a generous helping of baked tortilla chips.

8. Basil Pesto Stuffed Mushrooms

Serves: 10

Ingredients:

- 10 crimini mushrooms, washed, remove stems

For topping:

- 2 tablespoons butter, melted
- ¾ cup panko breadcrumbs
- 2 tablespoons fresh parsley, chopped

For filling:

- 1 cup fresh basil leaves, washed
- 1 tablespoon pumpkin seeds
- 4 cloves garlic, peeled, sliced
- ¼ teaspoon kosher salt
- 2 tablespoons fresh parmesan cheese, shredded
- ½ tablespoon olive oil
- 1 teaspoon lemon juice

Method:

1. Place mushroom caps on a baking sheet with the top side facing down (stem side should face up)
2. To make filling: Add basil, pumpkin seeds, cheese, garlic, and oil, salt and lemon juice into the food processor bowl. Pulse until it is well combined.
3. Fill a generous amount of this mixture into the mushroom caps.

4. To make topping: Mix together in a bowl, panko breadcrumbs, butter and parsley. Sprinkle this mixture over the filled mushroom caps.

5. Bake in a preheated oven at 350 F for 10-15 minutes or until the top is browned according to the way you like it.

9. Corn Tamales with Avocado Tomatillo Salsa

Serves: 3

Ingredients:

- 9 dried corn husks + extra to tie
- 1 cup masa harina (Spanish dough flour)
- ½ teaspoon baking powder
- ¼ cup lukewarm water
- ¼ teaspoon salt
- Red pepper flakes to taste
- 1 ½ cups fresh corn kernels or frozen corn kernels, thawed
- 2 tablespoons green bell pepper, chopped
- 2 tablespoons red bell pepper, chopped
- 1 ½ tablespoons canola oil
- 2 tablespoons yellow onion, diced

For the salsa:

- 2 tablespoons avocado, finely chopped
- 2 teaspoons fresh lime juice
- 1 small jalapeño, deseeded, minced
- 2 ½ ounces tomatillos, husked under warm running water, chopped
- 1 tablespoon fresh cilantro, chopped
- 1/8 teaspoon salt or to taste

Method:

1. Take a bowl of water and add the cornhusks. Let it soak in it for 10 minutes.
2. Discard the water and rinse the husk. Dry with a clean towel and set aside.
3. Add 1-¼ cups corn kernels into the food processor and pulse until it forms a coarse puree.
4. Transfer into a bowl. Add masa harina, lukewarm water, salt, baking powder and oil. Mix well with your hands.
5. Place a nonstick pan over medium heat. Add bell peppers, onion and ¼ cup corn kernels and sauté until the vegetables are crisp as well as tender.
6. Add red pepper flakes and stir. Remove from heat.
7. To make tamale: Place 9 soaked and dried cornhusk on your work area. Divide the masa mixture among the husks along the middle portion along the length. Place a tablespoon of the sautéed vegetables.
8. Fold the long sides of the husk over the filling. Fold the sides as well.
9. Make thin strips from the extra husk. Use this strip to fasten the filled husk.
10. Repeat with the remaining husks.
11. Place the tamale in a steamer basket and steam for 50-60 minutes.
12. Meanwhile make the salsa as follow: Add tomatillos, avocado, cilantro, lime juice, jalapeño and salt into a bowl. Toss well. Cover and set aside for a while for the flavors to set in.
13. Serve 3 tamales per serving with salsa.

10. Black Bean and Salmon Tostadas

Serves: 6

Ingredients:

- 12 corn tortillas (6 inches each)
- 1 ½ cans (6-7 ounces each) boneless, skinless wild Alaskan salmon, drained
- 3 tablespoons pickled jalapeños, minced
- 3 tablespoons pickling juice of the pickled jalapeños
- 3 tablespoons fresh cilantro, chopped
- 5 tablespoons low fat sour cream
- 1 large avocado, peeled, pitted, chopped
- 3 cups coleslaw mix or shredded cabbage
- 1 ½ cans (15 ounces each) black beans, rinsed
- 3 scallions, chopped
- Lime wedges to serve, optional
- 3 tablespoons prepared salsa
- Cooking spray

Method:

1. Place the oven racks in the upper and lower thirds in the oven.
2. Preheat the oven to 375 F.
3. Spray both sides of the tortillas with cooking spray.
4. Place 3 tortillas each on 2 baking sheets. If it is not fitting in, then bake in batches.
5. Bake for 12-14 minutes until light brown. Flip sides half way through baking.
6. Add salmon, jalapeños and avocado into a bowl.
7. Add cabbage or coleslaw mix, cilantro, minced pickle and pickling juice into another bowl.

8. Add black beans, salsa, sour cream and scallions into the food processor and pulse until smooth.
9. Transfer into a microwave safe bowl. Microwave on high until thoroughly heated.
10. To make tostadas: Place tortillas on your work area. Spread bean mixture on each.
11. Divide the salmon mixture over the bean mixture. Place cabbage mixture.
12. Serve the tostadas with lime wedges.

11. Gazpacho with Chickpeas

Serves: 3

Ingredients:

- 7.5 ounces canned chickpeas, rinsed, drained
- 8 cherry tomatoes, quartered
- 2 tablespoons red onion, chopped
- Hot pepper sauce to taste
- 2 tablespoons lime juice
- 3 cups vegetable juice, unsalted
- 1 small cucumber, deseeded, chopped
- 2 tablespoons fresh cilantro or parsley, chopped
- 1 clove garlic, minced
- 3 lime wedges

Method:

1. Add all the ingredients except lime into a bowl. Mix well.
2. Cover and place in the refrigerator for at least an hour for the flavors to set in.
3. Ladle into chilled soup bowls. Place a lime wedge in each bowl.
4. Serve right away.

Don't forget to like this book and leave a review here: https://www.amazon.com/DASH-Diet-Made-Easy-Beginners-ebook/dp/B071GRN2CV

12. Mango Salsa Pizza

Serves: 8

Ingredients:

- 1 medium red bell pepper, chopped
- 1 medium green bell pepper, chopped
- 1 cup mango, peeled, deseeded, chopped
- 1 cup onions, minced
- 1 cup pineapple tidbits
- 1 cup fresh cilantro, chopped
- 2 tablespoons lime juice
- 2 prepared whole grain pizza crusts (12 inches each)

Method:

1. Let the oven preheat to 425 F.
2. Take 2 round baking pans of 12 inches each. Grease with cooking spray.
3. Add all the ingredients except crust into a bowl and stir. Set aside until the pizza crust is ready.
4. Divide the dough into 2 equal portions. Roll each into a round of 12 inches and press it into the prepared baking pans.
5. Place the baking pans in batches in the oven and bake for 15 minutes.
6. Remove the crust from the oven. Divide the mango salsa over the crusts.
7. Place the crust back in the oven and bake for 7-10 minutes.
8. Slice into wedges.
9. Serve right away.

Chapter 4: DASH Diet Side Dish Recipes

13. Chicken Salad with Pineapple & Balsamic Vinegar

Serves: 4

Ingredients:

- 2 chicken breasts, skinless, boneless, cut into cubes
- 4 ounces unsweetened pineapple chunks
- 2 tablespoons pineapple juice or juice of the canned pineapple chunks
- 2 cups fresh baby spinach leaves
- 1 cup broccoli florets
- 1 medium red onion, thinly sliced
- 2 teaspoons olive oil

For the vinaigrette:

- 2 tablespoons olive oil
- 1 teaspoon sugar
- 1 tablespoon balsamic vinegar
- A large pinch ground cinnamon

Method:

1. To make vinaigrette: Add olive oil, sugar, pineapple juice, vinegar and cinnamon into a bowl. Whisk until well combined. Set aside for a while for the flavors to set in.
2. Place a nonstick pan over medium heat. Add olive oil. When the oil is heated, add chicken and sauté until brown.

3. Transfer into a bowl. Add remaining salad ingredients. Toss well and set aside.
4. Pour the dressing over the salad. Toss well.
5. Serve right away.

14. Spicy Roasted Broccoli

Serves: 4

Ingredients:

- 4 cups broccoli, cut into 2 inch pieces
- ¼ teaspoon salt free seasoning blend
- 2 cloves garlic, peeled, minced
- 2 tablespoons olive oil, divided
- Freshly ground pepper to taste
- 1/8 teaspoon crushed red pepper flakes

Method:

1. Let the oven preheat to 450 F.
2. Add broccoli into a bowl. Pour 1-tablespoon olive oil over it and toss well.
3. Season with pepper and salt free seasoning. Place the seasoned broccoli on a rimmed baking sheet.
4. Place in the oven and roast for 15 minutes.
5. Meanwhile, add garlic, red pepper flakes and 1-tablespoon olive oil into a bowl. Mix well and pour over the broccoli. Toss well.
6. Roast for 8-10 minutes or until the broccoli begins to turn brown.
7. Serve hot.

15. Brown Rice Pilaf with Asparagus and Mushrooms

Serves: 3

Ingredients:

- ½ tablespoon olive oil
- 1 ½ cups water
- ½ cup brown rice
- ½ teaspoon low sodium chicken flavored bouillon granules
- ¼ pound fresh mushrooms, thinly sliced
- ¼ pound asparagus tips
- ¼ cup fresh parsley, chopped
- 1 small onion, chopped
- A large pinch ground nutmeg
- 1-2 tablespoons Swiss cheese, finely grated

Method:

1. Place a saucepan over medium heat. Add olive oil. When the oil is heated, add rice and sauté until the rice is toasted and slightly golden brown in color.
2. Pour water. Add bouillon granules, mushrooms, onion and nutmeg and stir. Bring to the boil.
3. Lower heat. Cover with a lid. Simmer until the rice is tender and cooked. Add more water if required.
4. Meanwhile, discard the hard stems of the asparagus. Chop into 1-inch pieces.
5. Add asparagus. Stir and cover again.
6. Cook for 4-5 minutes. Add cheese and stir.
7. Sprinkle parsley and serve right away.

16. Holiday Green Bean Casserole

Serves: 5

Ingredients:

- 2 teaspoons olive oil, divided
- 2 tablespoons onions, finely chopped
- 1 medium onion, thinly sliced
- 1 clove garlic, finely chopped
- 1 cup mushrooms, sliced
- 1 tablespoon water
- 1 ½ tablespoons flour
- ¾ cup skim milk
- ¼ teaspoon dried ground thyme
- ¼ cup fresh whole wheat bread crumbs
- ½ pound fresh green beans, trimmed, cut into 1 inch pieces

Method:

1. Let the oven preheat to 350 F.
2. Place a skillet over low heat. Add 1-teaspoon olive oil. When the oil is heated, add sliced onions and cook until the onions are golden brown in color. Remove the onions with a slotted spoon and set aside in a bowl.
3. Add 1-teaspoon olive oil into the skillet. Add chopped onion and garlic and sauté for 2 – 3 minutes. Add water and mushrooms and cook for 4-5 minutes.
4. Sprinkle flour and thyme over the mushroom mixture. Mix well.
5. Slowly pour in the milk. Stir constantly.
6. Raise the heat to medium and cook until the sauce becomes thick in consistency.

7. Remove from heat. Cover with a lid and set aside for a while until the beans is cooked.

8. Place a saucepan with water over medium heat. Bring to the boil. Add beans and cook until the beans are tender. Drain the beans in a colander.

9. Grease an ovenproof casserole dish with cooking spray. Spread the green beans in it.

10. Spread the mushroom mixture over the beans. Sprinkle the browned onions and finally with the breadcrumbs.

11. Bake until the top is golden brown in color.

Chapter 5: DASH Diet Dinner Recipes

17. Millet Stuffed Peppers with Ginger and Tofu

Serves: 8

Ingredients:

- 1 ½ cups millet
- 3 ½ cups water
- 8 ounces flavored, baked tofu, diced
- ½ cup fresh cilantro, chopped
- 3 tablespoons low sodium tamari
- 2 cloves garlic, minced
- 2 teaspoons sugar
- 4 large red bell peppers, halved lengthwise, deseeded
- 4 medium carrots, grated
- 6 tablespoons canola oil
- 4 teaspoons Serrano pepper or jalapeño pepper, minced
- 2 teaspoons fresh ginger, grated

Method:

1. Place the rack of the oven in the upper third part of the oven.
2. Let the oven preheat to 425 F.
3. Place a saucepan with water and millet over high heat. Bring to the boil.
4. Lower heat and cover with a lid. Simmer until the millets are tender and all the water is absorbed. Turn off the heat.

5. Place the bell peppers in a broiler safe dish with the cut side up.

6. Place the dish in the oven and bake for 6-8 minutes until slightly soft. Remove from the oven and increase the broiler heat to high.

7. Add rest of the ingredients into a large bowl. Add millets and stir. Divide the mixture among the bell pepper halves.

8. Place the dish with the peppers in the oven and broil for 4-6 minutes.

18. Orange and Pistachio Crusted Pork Tenderloin

Serves: 8

Ingredients:

- 1 cup pearl barley, rinsed
- 6 cups water
- 1 ½ teaspoons salt, divided
- 4 large cloves garlic
- 2 pounds pork tenderloin, trimmed
- 6 tablespoons orange marmalade
- 4 teaspoons lemon zest
- 2/3 cup shelled pistachio, toasted
- 1 teaspoon pepper powder, divided
- 4 tablespoons extra virgin olive oil, divided
- 3 pounds green beans, trimmed
- 1 cup wild rice

Method:

1. Add rice, barley, water and ½ teaspoon salt into a large saucepan. Place the saucepan over medium heat. Bring to the boil.
2. Lower heat and cover the saucepan with a lid. Simmer until tender (it should not be too soft). It should take about 45-60 minutes.
3. Place oven rack in the center and bottom third position. Let the oven preheat to 450 F.
4. Add pistachio and garlic into the small jar of the food processor. Pulse until it is finely chopped.
5. Sprinkle pork with ½ teaspoon salt and ½ teaspoon pepper.

6. Place an ovenproof skillet over medium high heat. Add 2 tablespoons olive oil. When the oil is heated, add pork and cook until brown all over. Turn off the heat.
7. Brush pork with marmalade. Next dredge in pistachio nuts. Place the pork in the same skillet.
8. Place the skillet on the center rack in the oven. Cook until done. When done, the internal temperature of the pork should be 145 F.
9. Remove the pork and place on your cutting board. When cool enough to handle, slice the pork carefully so that the crust does not fall off.
10. Meanwhile, add beans into a large bowl. Pour remaining oil on it. Toss well and transfer on a rimmed baking sheet.
11. Place the baking sheet on the bottom third rack in the oven. Bake until the beans are crisp as well as tender.
12. Serve crusted pork with cooked barley and wild rice along with green beans.

19. Chicken Brats

Serves: 3

Ingredients:

- ½ cup yellow onion, minced
- ½ teaspoon canola oil
- ½ pound ground chicken breast
- ½ teaspoon cumin seeds
- ¼ teaspoon white pepper powder
- ½ teaspoon black pepper powder
- ¼ teaspoon cayenne pepper
- 1/8 teaspoon ground nutmeg
- ½ teaspoon celery seeds
- 2 cloves garlic, minced
- ½ cup cooked brown rice
- 1 teaspoon fennel seeds
- ½ teaspoon paprika
- ½ teaspoon fresh rosemary, minced
- ½ teaspoon ground mustard seeds

Method:

1. Place a skillet over medium heat. Add oil. When the oil is heated, add onion and garlic and sauté until brown.
2. Remove from heat. Add rest of the ingredients. Mix well. Transfer into a bowl.
3. Cover and place in the refrigerator for an hour.
4. Divide the mixture into 3 equal portions. Shape each into a sausage.
5. Place on a baking sheet.
6. Bake in a preheated oven at 350 F for about 10 minutes or until the internal temperature shows 125 F.

7. Refrigerate until use.
8. To use: Grill on a preheated grill and serve with rolls or a salad or side dish of your choice.

20. Homestyle Turkey Soup

Serves: 5

Ingredients:

For broth:

- ½ turkey carcass
- 4 cups low sodium chicken broth
- 2 cups water
- 3 medium onions, quartered
- 3 medium onions, chopped

For soup:

- 1 medium onion, chopped
- ½ cup celery, chopped
- 2 carrots, peeled, cut into thin strips
- A large pinch dried thyme
- Black pepper to taste
- 7 ounces canned tomatoes, unsalted
- ¼ pound left over light turkey meat, cut into bite size pieces
- ½ cup rutabaga or turnip, peeled, diced
- 2 tablespoons fresh parsley, chopped
- 1 bay leaf
- 2 tablespoons pearl barley, uncooked
- 8 ounces canned white beans, drained, rinsed

Method:

1. To make stock: Add turkey carcass, water, broth and onions into a soup pot.

2. Place the pot over high heat. Bring to the boil. Lower heat and cover with a lid.
3. Simmer for about 30-45 minutes. Strain the stock and discard the solids. Pour the stock back into the pot.
4. Add all the ingredients of the soup into the pot. Place the pot over high heat and bring to the boil.
5. Lower heat and cover with a lid. Simmer for 45-60 minutes.
6. Ladle into soup bowls and serve with crusty bread.

21. Easy Roasted Salmon

Serves: 2

Ingredients:

- 2 wild salmon fillets (6 ounces each)
- Freshly ground black pepper to taste
- 2 cloves garlic, minced
- 2 tablespoons lemon juice
- 2 tablespoons fresh dill, minced

Method:

1. Grease a baking dish with cooking spray. Place salmon fillets in it.
2. Drizzle lemon juice on it. Sprinkle pepper, garlic and dill.
3. Place the dish in a preheated oven and bake at 400 F for 20-22 minutes or until the salmon is opaque in the center.

Chapter 6: DASH Diet Dessert Recipes

22. Healthy Chocolate Pudding

Serves: 8

Ingredients:

- 3 cups vanilla soy milk, unsweetened
- 2 medium bananas, peeled, sliced
- 1 large ripe avocado, peeled, pitted, chopped
- 4 packets splenda or stevia drops to taste
- ½ cup cocoa powder, unsweetened
- ½ cup almonds or walnuts, chopped

Method:

1. Add all the ingredients into a blender and blend until smooth.
2. Pour into dessert bowls. Chill for a few hours and serve.

23. Peach Floats

Serves: 2

Ingredients:

- 7 ½ ounces canned peaches, drain most of the juice, mashed
- 16 ounces club soda or seltzer water
- A pinch ground nutmeg
- 2 cups vanilla ice milk
- ¼ cup low fat whipped topping

Method:

1. Divide the peach into 2 tall glasses. Pour 2 tablespoons peach juice into each glass.
2. Add a cup of milk into each glass. Divide and pour the soda in the glasses.
3. Top with whipped topping. Sprinkle nutmeg on top and serve.

24. Grapes and Walnuts with Lemon Sour cream

Serves: 3

Ingredients:

- ¼ cup fat free sour cream
- ¼ teaspoon lemon zest, grated
- 1/8 teaspoon vanilla extract
- ¾ cup seedless green grapes
- ¾ cup seedless red grapes
- 2 tablespoons walnuts
- 1 tablespoon powdered sugar
- ¼ teaspoon lemon juice

Method:

1. To make lemon sour cream: Add sugar, sour cream, vanilla, lemon juice and zest into a bowl. Whisk well. Cover and refrigerate for 5-6 hours.
2. Divide the red and green grapes among 3 dessert bowls. Drizzle lemon sour cream on top. Garnish with walnuts and serve.

25. Creamy Fruit Dessert

Serves: 2

Ingredients:

- 2 ounces fat free cream cheese, softened
- ½ teaspoon sugar
- 5.5 ounces canned mandarin oranges, drained
- 4 ounces canned water packed pineapple chunks, drained
- 4 ounces canned water packed peach slices, drained
- 2 tablespoons shredded coconut, toasted
- ¼ cup plain fat free yogurt
- ¼ teaspoon vanilla extract

Method:

1. Whisk together with an electric mixer (on high speed), cream cheese, sugar, vanilla and yogurt until smooth.
2. Transfer into a bowl. Add the fruits and stir. Chill for a few hours.
3. Serve garnished with coconut.

Conclusion

With that, sweet one, we have come to the end of this book.

I am sure you can hardly wait to try these recipes and get started to bring about a change in your diet and lifestyle. You don't have to restrict yourself to these ingredients, as long as you restrict yourself to using DASH compliant ingredients and control your sodium intake.

I wish to thank you once again for choosing this book! Good luck!

Don't forget to like this book and leave a review here: https://www.amazon.com/DASH-Diet-Made-Easy-Beginners-ebook/dp/B071GRN2CV

Check Out My Other Books

Below you'll find another one of my popular books that. Simply search for the title on the Amazon website or click on the title!

Care Less, Live More: How to Stop Giving a You Know What

Diabetic Smoothie Recipes: 35 Easy & Delicious Smoothie Recipes for Diabetics